I0820722

A LITTLE BOOK *of* SELF-CARE *for* CAREGIVERS

A LITTLE BOOK *of* SELF-CARE *for* CAREGIVERS

with a foreword by

BEVERLY E. THORN, PHD

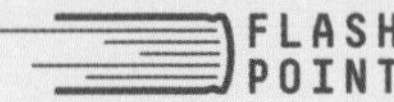

Published by Flashpoint™ Books, Seattle
www.flashpointbooks.com

Produced by Girl Friday Productions

Design: Rachel Marek
Development & editorial: Sara Spees Addicott
Production editorial: Reshma Kooner

Image credits (all credits belong to Shutterstock users): front cover (teacup), Le Panda; back cover, 79, 124, Artnizu; front cover, iii, TWINS DESIGN STUDIO; vii, Inna Sinano; 3, 20, 24, 44, 98, My Ho; 4, Yuliia Druzenko; 6, Atomorfen Illustration; 9, Lisa Art; 10, Annet Kuzmina; 13, 17, Astaru; 14–15, one AND only; 19, 71, chyworks; 27, mimibubu; 28–29, 95, Joann Vector Artist; 30, 77, Anastasia Lembrik; 33, 47, Daria Ustiugova; 34, 35, Mika Besfamilnaya; 36, Natali Mias; 39, Yulia Bikirova; 43, lacuarela; 49, 59, 114, Palm Stocker; 53, Liska Art; 56, VectorDecor; 61, briget durich; 62, medelwardi20; 65, K.BOM; 67, pixachew; 68, Nancy White; 74, lichu; 80, 128, Magician ART; 82, 83, abusyahna; 87, Eva Kleinman; 88, Anna Hnatiuk; 92, Onesweetlime; 97, Olga Maha; 102, Cat_arch_angel; 105, Eva Kleinman; 106, Nataliia K; 111, Iya Balushkina; 117, Eisfrei; 118, Nanya; 122, Ermakova Marina

ISBN (hardcover): 978-1-954854-38-3
ISBN (ebook): 978-1-954854-41-3

Library of Congress Control Number: 2025933978

Printed in China

First edition

The information provided in this book is for educational purposes only. It is not a substitute for professional medical advice. If you are experiencing potential physical issues or having thoughts of self-harm, reach out to a trusted individual so they can help you find appropriate care.

"The closest thing to
being cared for is to care
for someone else."

—Carson McCullers

FOREWORD

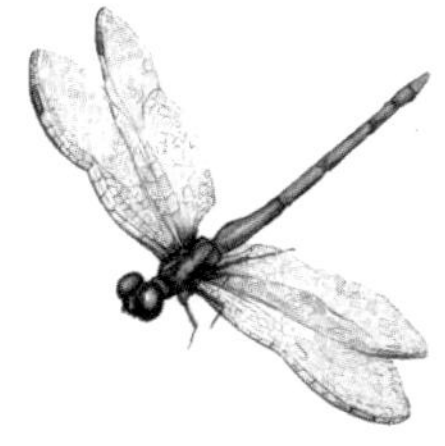

Have you ever been told that you need to take care of yourself, as if all you needed was a reminder and you'd be off on the next Caribbean cruise? Of course those of us who enlist in caregiving want to center our own well-being, too, but the prospect of doing so can feel daunting—almost insurmountable. How do we make time for ourselves when there's so much to do for the person we love? Who do those doing the supporting turn to for support?

This book focuses on care for the caregiver, and as such, it is revolutionary in its purpose. Traditionally, the caregiver has tended to fade into the background, their well-being given less emphasis, possibly because the person who is ill, injured, or struggling has obvious, often visible needs. When I became a full-time caregiver for my husband with dementia, I moved from being a psychologist helping patients cope with chronic illness and pain to being one of the multitude of people caring for a loved one. It was different, and it was humbling. Caregiver needs may not be as obvious, but they are just as essential. As a caregiver, it is not simply important to care for ourselves so that we can be "up to the task" of caring for our loved one; we care for ourselves because we are individuals worthy of love, honor, and self-care in our own right.

Though caregiving can feel lonely, you are not alone. In fact, you are part of a mighty army and form the backbone of care for millions of people around the world. And the first step to caring for yourself needn't be a complete upending of your caregiving relationship. Rather, it can be bite-size—knowing that it's okay to take a moment now and then to connect with your own emotions, needs, desires, and sense of self. Microdoses of self-care can pave the way to a consistent practice that contributes to your strength and resilience in even the most difficult times.

Self-care is not selfish. It is your lifeline. I hope you can find strength, hope, and little gems of inspiration in this book. Remember: You are worthy of care just because you are you.

—Beverly E. Thorn, PhD, author of
Before I Lose My Own Mind: Navigating Life as a Dementia Caregiver

INTRODUCTION

Caregiving can be a lonely road. It's an honor and a privilege—but one that often involves a million invisible tasks, worries, and thoughts pulling you in different directions. We know caregiving comes from the heart, and caregivers aren't looking for credit, but the book you're holding in your hands is a reminder that *you* matter. Not just the work you're doing, but your own emotional and physical well-being. Caregivers need care, too—the occasional recognition of your hard and important work, a deep breath, a hug, a few kind words, or a laugh.

There are so many ways you may be called upon to serve a loved one in need, and maybe you never expected it. You might be caring for a parent, spouse, child, sibling, or beloved friend. The role you play as a caregiver will vary, of course, depending on who you're caring for—and what type of care they need. Nursing someone back to health from surgery is different from ministering to someone with a chronic condition, or a person at the end of their life. Tangling with memory-care issues will be fundamentally different from helping a child with a broken leg or a friend suffering from a mental health crisis. So, too, will be the experience of the person receiving your care and what their relationship with you looks like. You might need to provide logistical help, emotional support, and physical assistance—sometimes all at once. You may be coordinating medical care for someone, trying to bring good cheer to a person who's feeling isolated and vulnerable, or attempting to put a brave face on for a difficult situation. You'll need to be nimble and strong and show up with an open heart. It can be *exhausting.*

Caregiving can take so many forms, but regardless of your situation, it is often a marathon, not a sprint. The trick is finding a balance between supporting your person the way you want to while also sustaining yourself. Taking care of yourself is not selfish; it's essential to providing the best care you can. This book gives you the tools to find the small wins that allow you to bring your very best and most joyful self to this role. We hope it buoys your spirits, helps you with a tip or two, and reminds you that this work you're doing is for your loved one. It matters.

Let the thoughts and affirmations contained here be a balm when you're feeling spent and the strategies to recharge your batteries spur you to action, so you can bring your best self to your person. Caregiving is an act of love and commitment—and courage. You've got this.

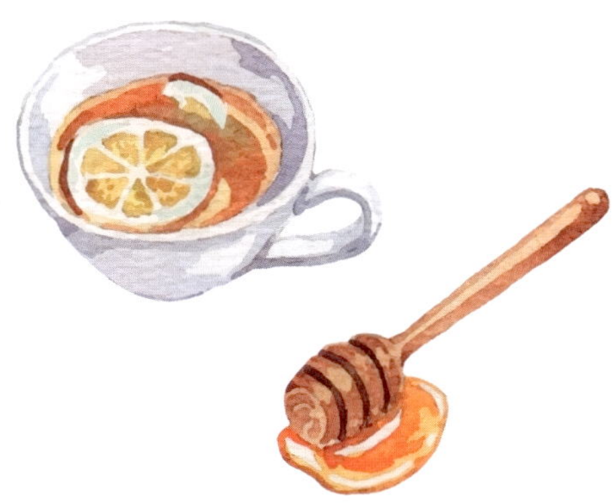

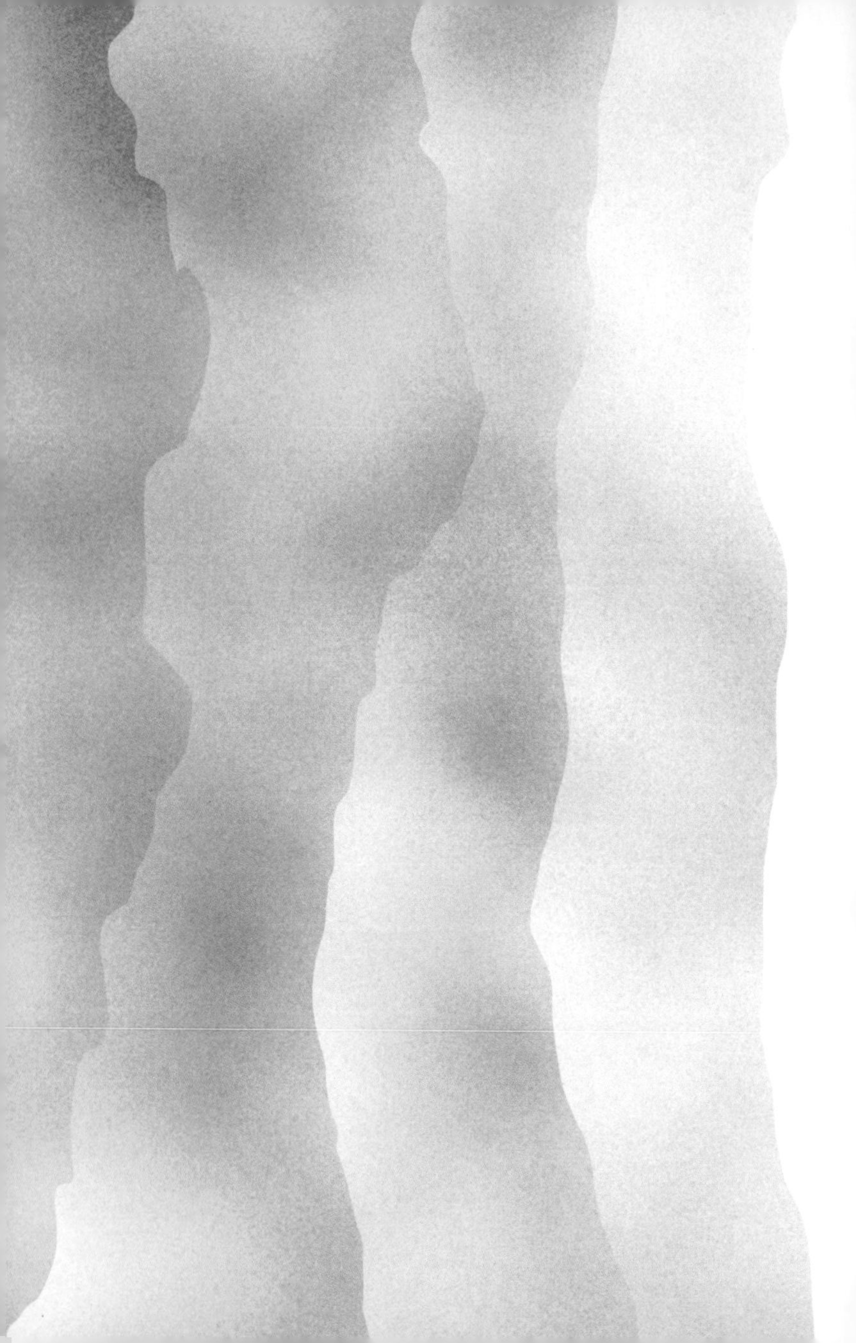

"I like to say that there are only four kinds of people in the world—those who have been caregivers, those who are currently caregivers, those who will be caregivers, and those who will need caregivers."

—Rosalynn Carter

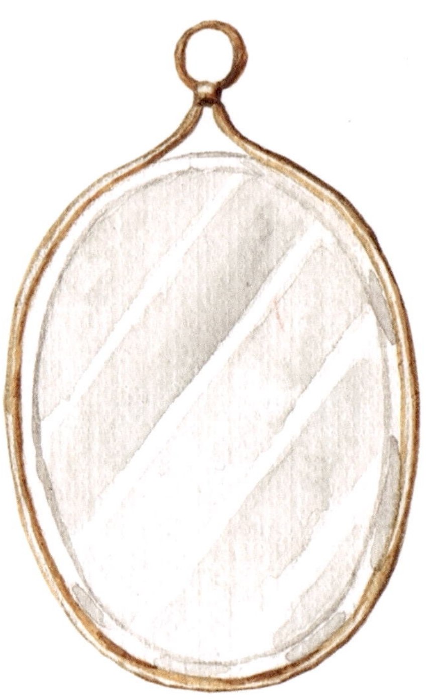

It is okay—and necessary—
to look after yourself, too.

Getting outside makes everything better. Mind, body, and soul.

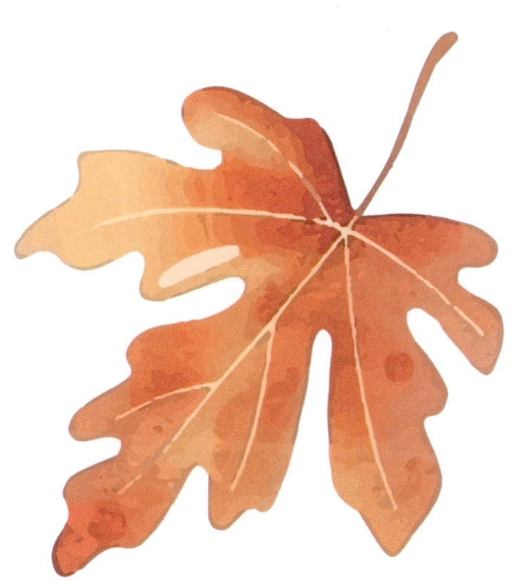

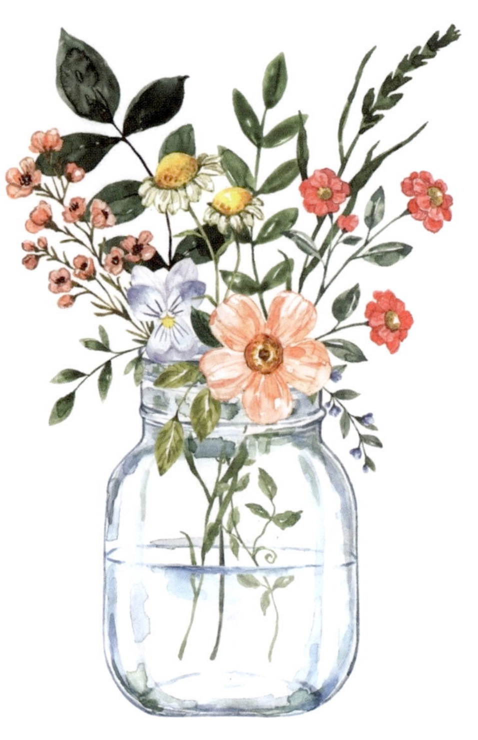

Small acts of self-care can make a world of difference. The cup of hot cocoa. The warm bath. The chat with a friend. The bouquet of flowers.

Caregiving is not either/or.
You need to take care of your
person *and* yourself.

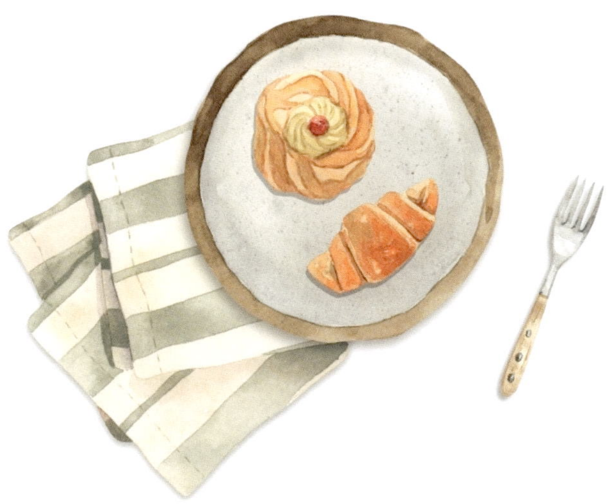

Sleep.

It will make everything
feel more possible.

Turn the music up and dance
out the stress in your kitchen
while you're making dinner.

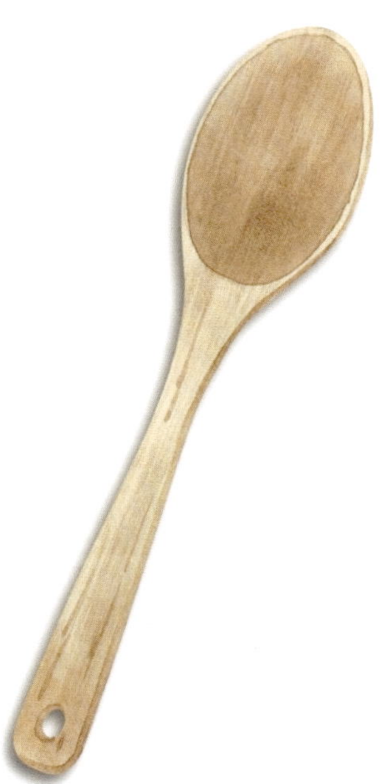

affirmation

SAY THIS OUT LOUD:

I have the resilience, strength,
and courage to face hard things.

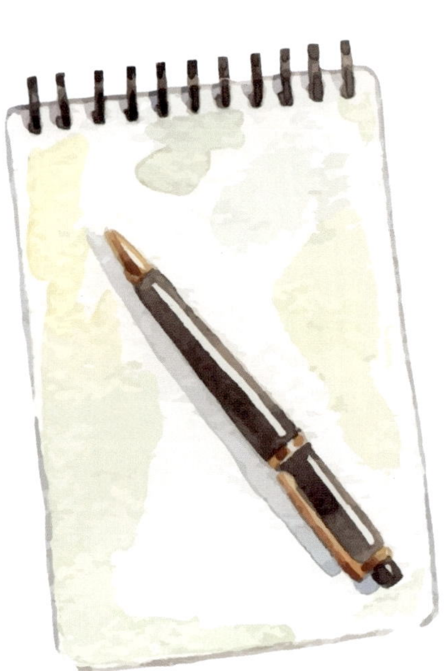

Take a look at community resources in your area that you might be able to use, such as occasional in-home nursing assistance or respite care. Start by asking your local hospital for their recommendations.

Simplify.

Perfection is overrated.

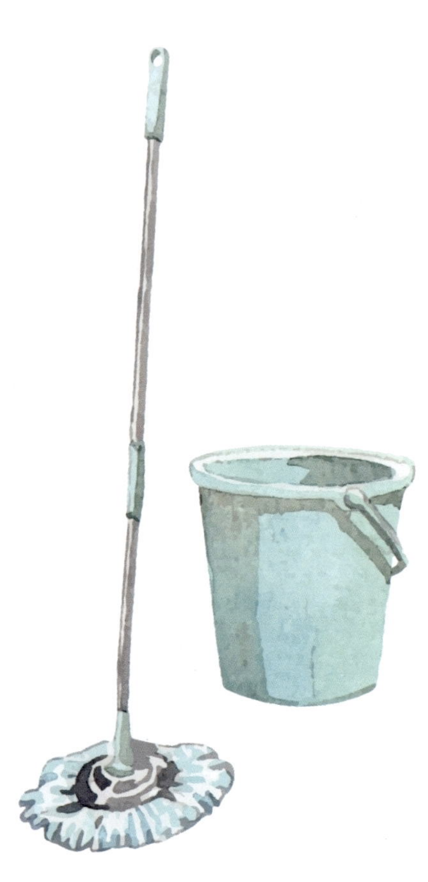

Build your village and let your people help you. Keep a list of small tasks and give people a choice when they ask how they can help. Yes, people really do want to help. They just don't know how.

Ask a friend to set up an online resource to help you request—and get!—the help you really need. CaringBridge and Caring Village are two examples.

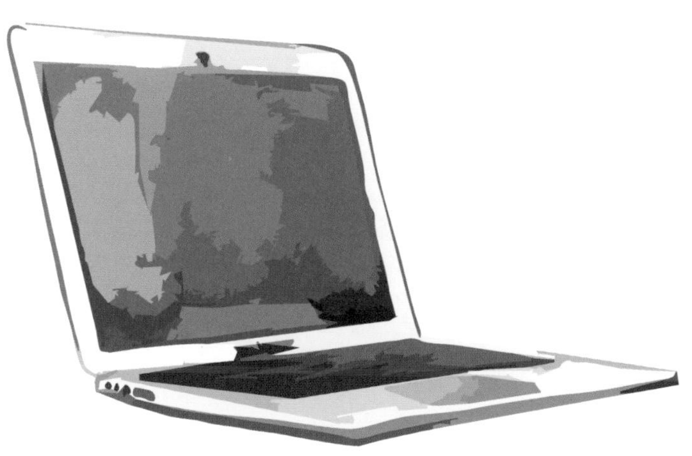

"Quality of life is determined by the person living it. Do for others not what you would do for yourself but what you think *they* would want."

—Penny Hawkins Smith, RN

@hospicenursepenny

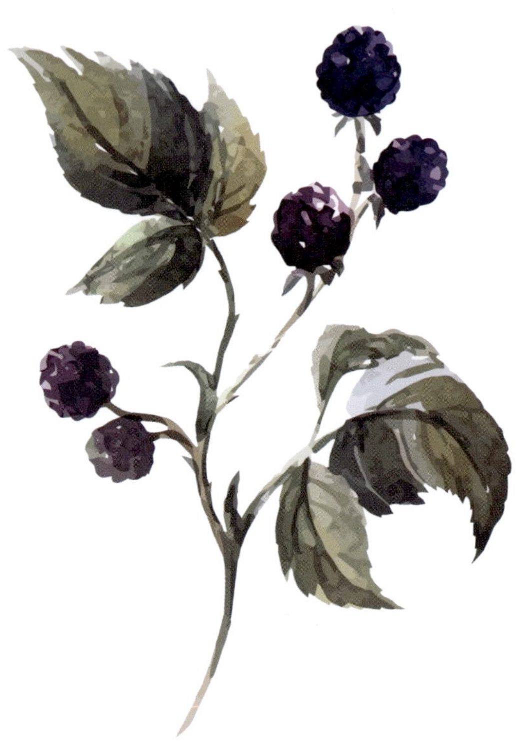

Forgive yourself any unkind thoughts. They happen, and they don't reflect the full truth of your relationship.

Remember the things *you* love to do. Bake those cookies. Plant that herb garden.

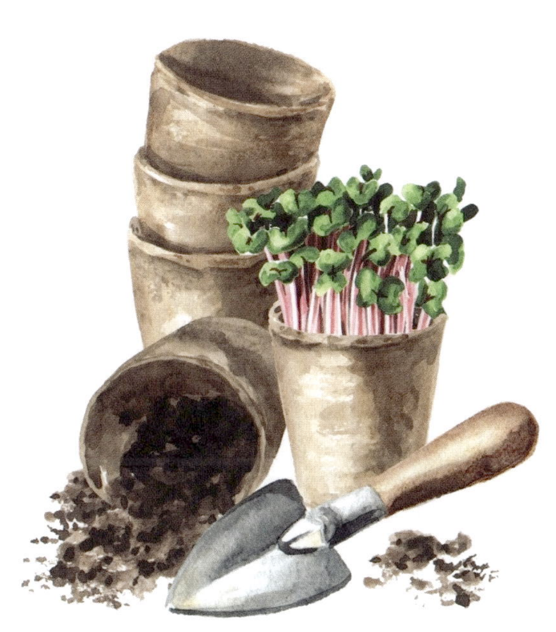

affirmation

SAY THIS OUT LOUD:

I am generous with myself
and my loved ones.

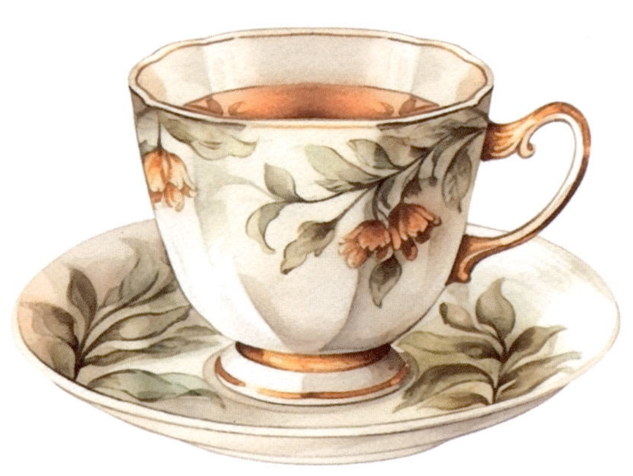

Embrace small rituals to ground you and maintain your equilibrium. Start your day with a morning walk or stretch. Write in a journal. Make that cup of tea in your favorite mug.

Butterflies rest when it rains because the water damages their wings. It's okay to rest during the storms of life. You'll fly again.

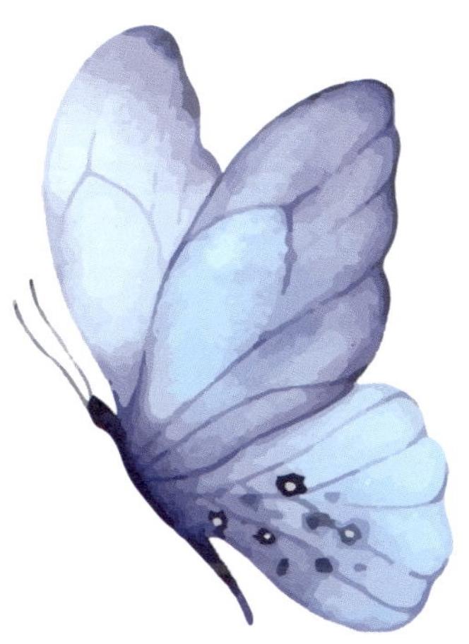

It’s okay to not be
strong all the time.

Cry. Vent. Feel. It's very likely you'll feel better afterward.

Love is tender. Love is kind. It's also fierce and determined and powerful.

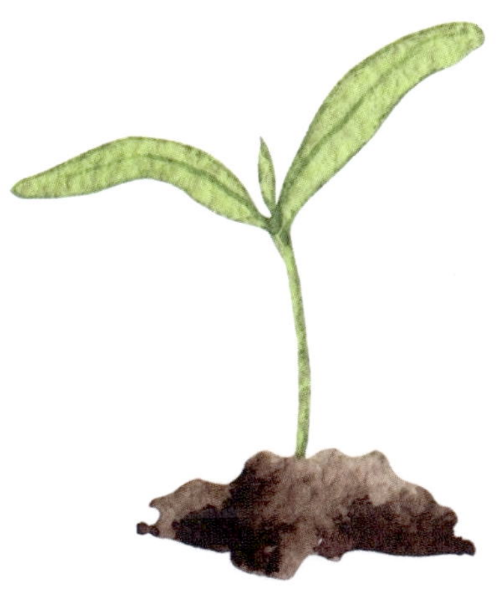

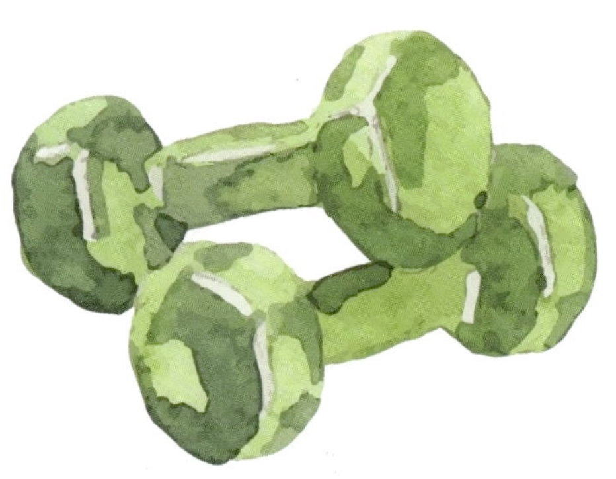

Find ways to let the feelings out. Talk to a trusted friend. Write them down. Sweat them out. Just don't keep them all bottled up inside.

Drink a full glass of cold water.

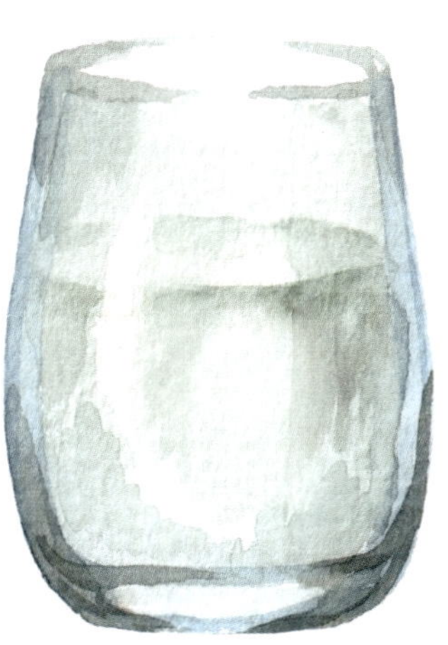

affirmation

SAY THIS OUT LOUD:

I am a caregiver, but I am other things, too. My interests and talents are valuable.

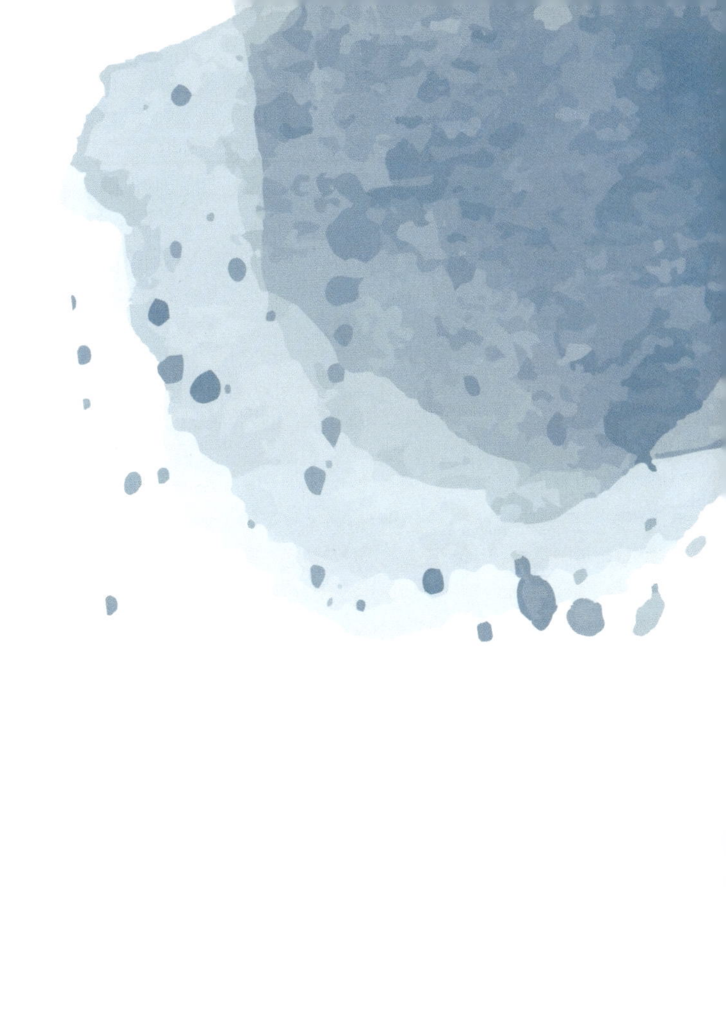

You are stronger
than you think.

Caregiving will test you, change you, and expand you, whether you want it to or not. Try to accept and not fight the change.

"I have found that the happiest people are those who do the most for others—the most miserable are those who do the least."

—Booker T. Washington

Focus on the small wins.

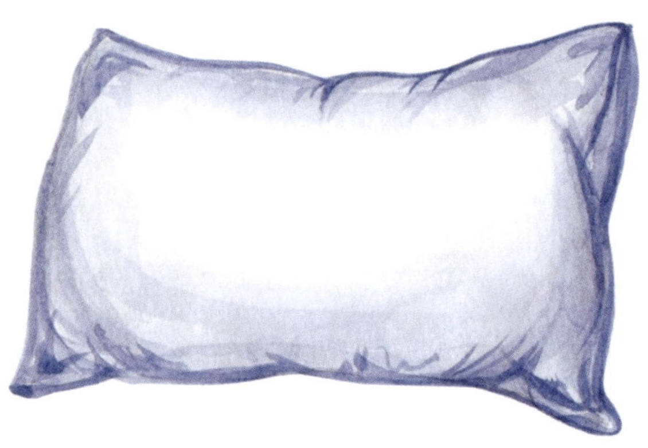

Lie down on your bed and close your eyes. Focus on relaxing each part of your body in turn, from your toes to your head. Breathe deeply.

Can't deal? Pause. Regroup.
Scroll through kitten memes or
videos of babies belly-laughing.

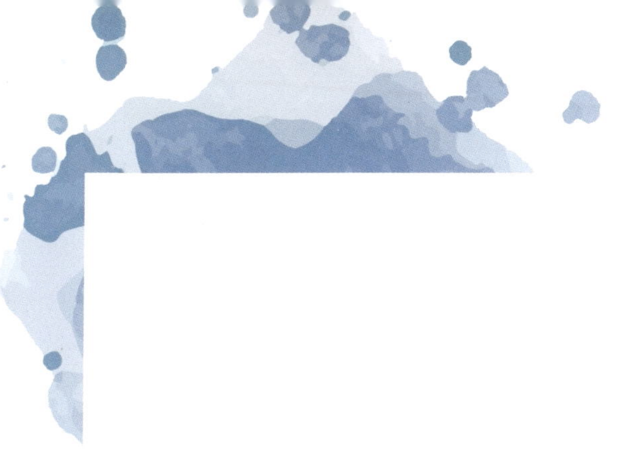

“A good laugh and a
long sleep are the two best
cures for anything.”

—Irish proverb

Caregiving is full of challenges,
but it may also open your eyes
to what really matters in life.
Be prepared to let in the good.

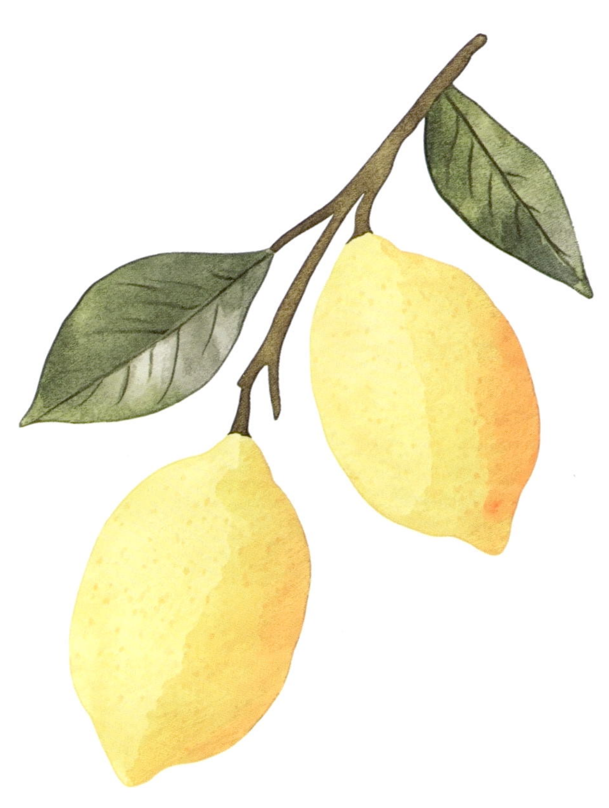

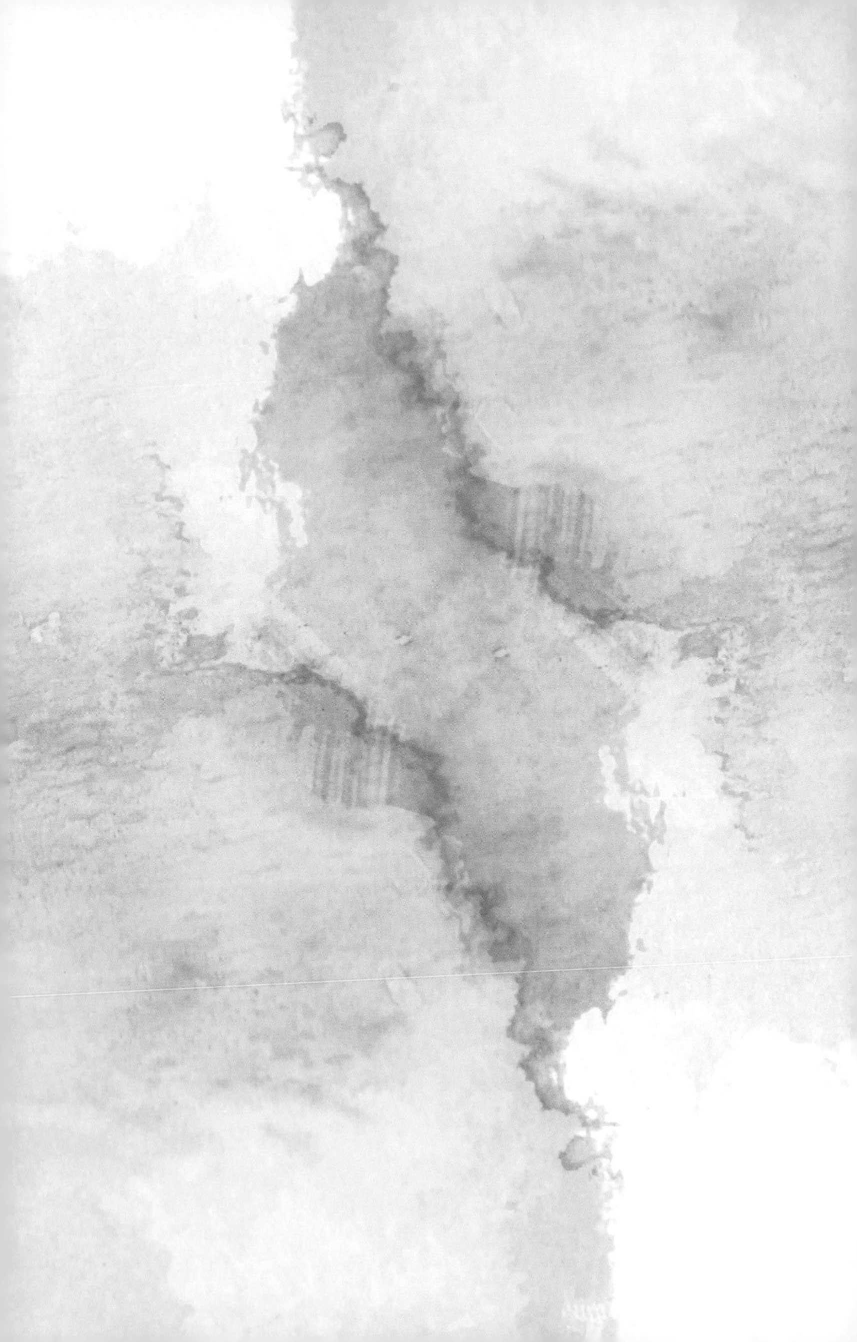

Find a support group. There is so much strength to be found in being heard, seen, and understood by someone who has walked in your shoes.

affirmation

SAY THIS OUT LOUD:

Even when I can't
see it, my loving care is
making a difference.

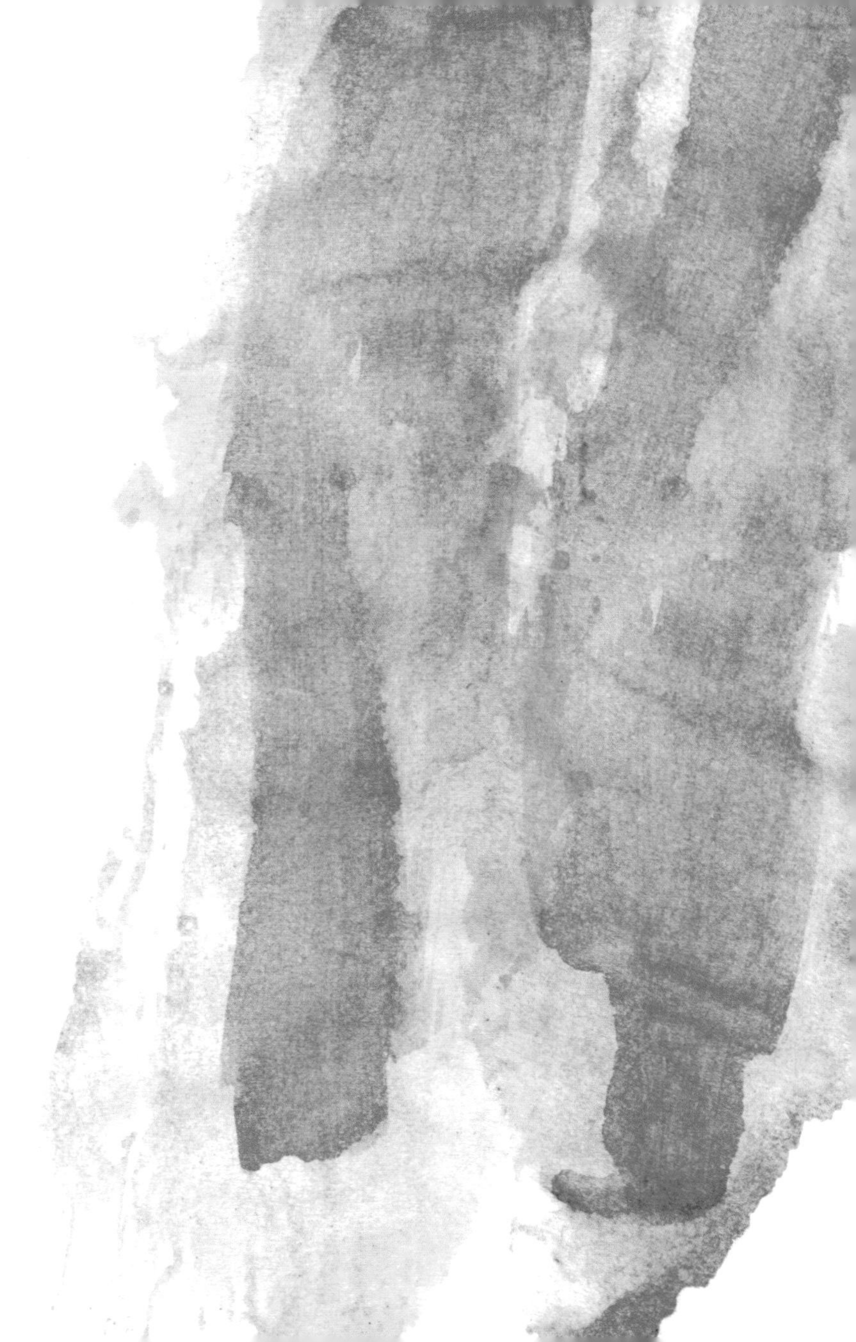

Sometimes you just need
to binge-watch that familiar
old show with all your
favorite characters who
seem like old friends.

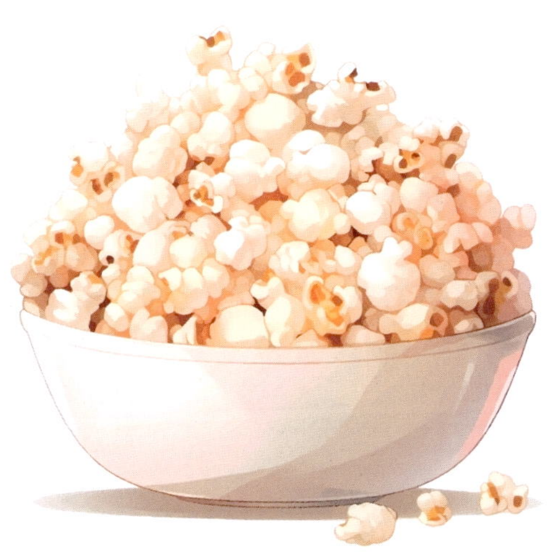

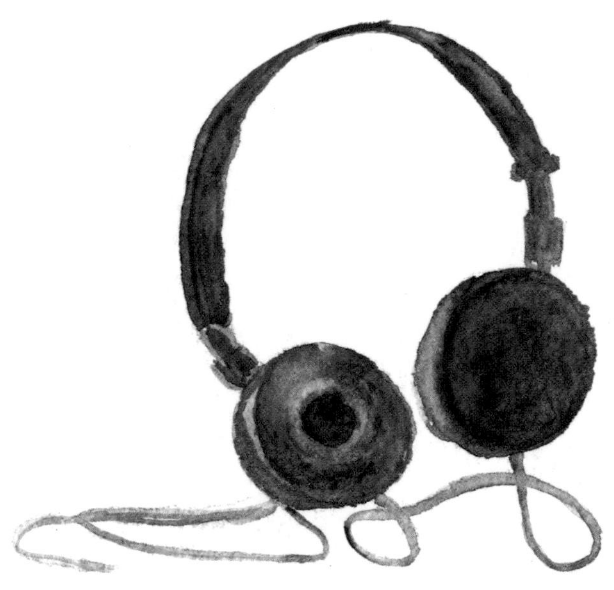

Audiobooks and podcasts offer a chance to learn, explore, or escape—even when you're too busy or tired to crack open a book.

Your best on any given day
is the best you have that
day. Showing up is what
matters, and that is enough.

"Caregiving often calls
us to lean into love we
didn't know possible."

—Tia Walker

Ask a friend to set up a meal train for you so you don't have to think about dinner every night.

You can decide whether you want folks to stop by and visit or just drop food off at the door.

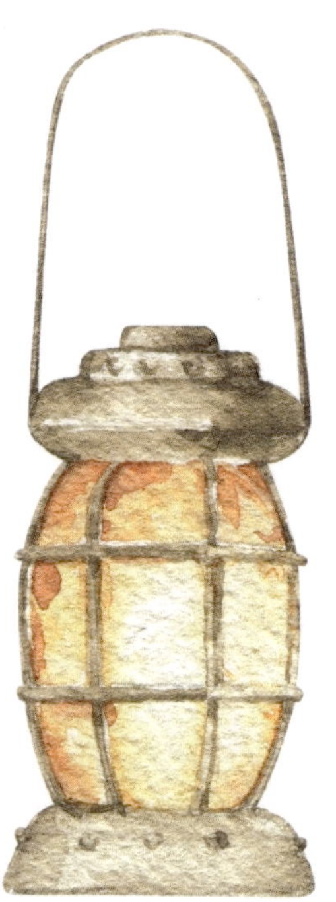

Let compassion be your guiding light—for the person you love and for yourself.

Play your favorite song at full volume. Sing in the car.

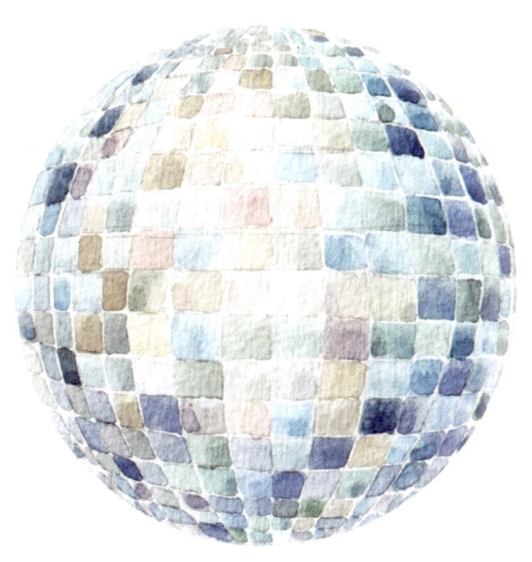

affirmation

SAY THIS OUT LOUD:

Even in difficult times,
I will find moments of
connection and joy.

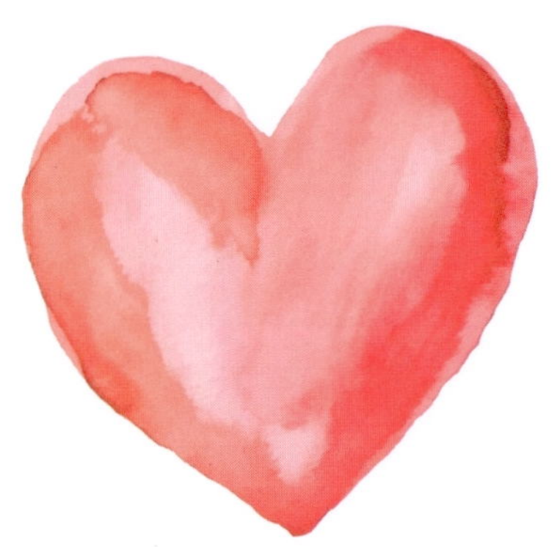

That long to-do list? It's love in action, every single line of it.

Try a breathing exercise, like box breathing. Breathe in through your nose for four seconds, hold it for four seconds, then breathe out through your mouth for four seconds.

Repeat ten times, and
feel your body relax.

"Where there is great love
there are always miracles."

—Willa Cather

Be on the lookout for glimmers. What is a glimmer, you ask? A tiny moment of joy, connection, or calm. They may be fleeting, but they are a balm for mind, body, and soul.

If you're struggling with asking for help, imagine that a friend or loved one is asking *you* for help. You'd help them, right? So take the leap and accept the help that's offered.

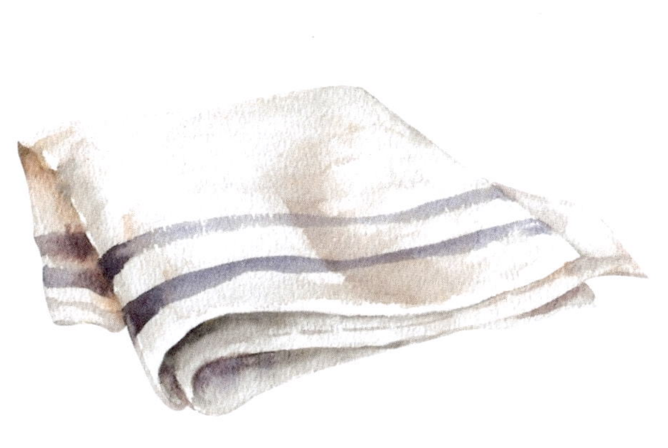

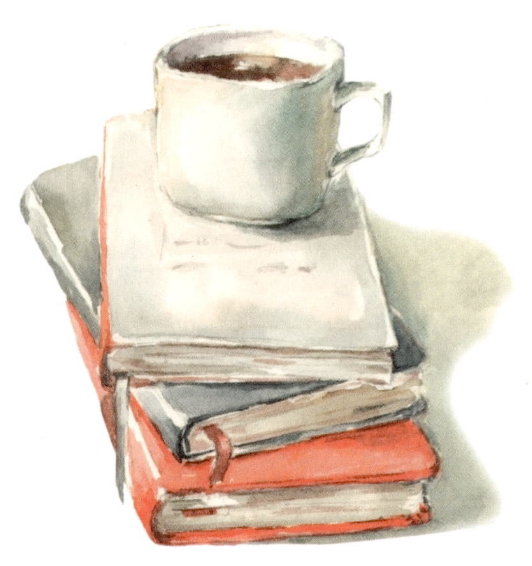

Ask if your person would like to be read to. Reading aloud to someone is also reading for yourself.

Things can feel harder
and scarier in the
middle of the night.

As the sun rises, so does the possibility of a better day.

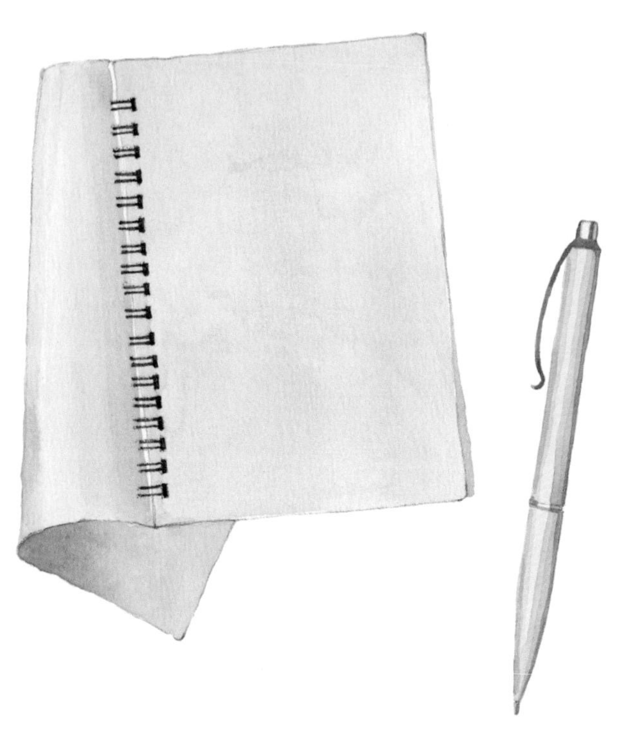

Keep a notebook by your bedside. That way, if something occurs to you in the middle of the night, you can jot it down and then give your mind permission to forget it and go back to sleep.

affirmation

SAY THIS OUT LOUD:

My presence matters.

If at all possible, delegate. Even if it means delegating dinner for yourself. Have food delivered to take something off your plate (and get something delicious onto your plate!).

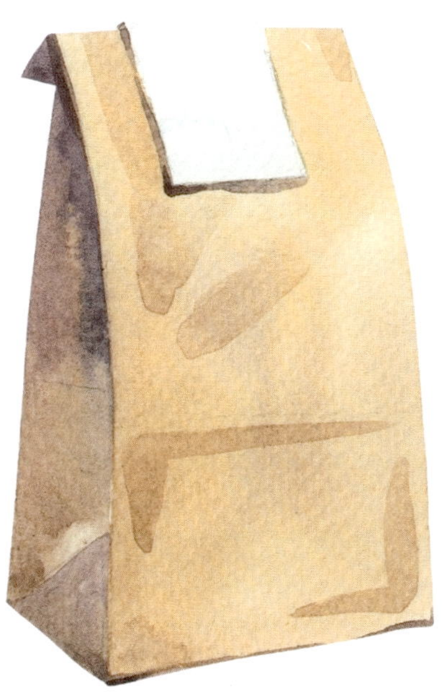

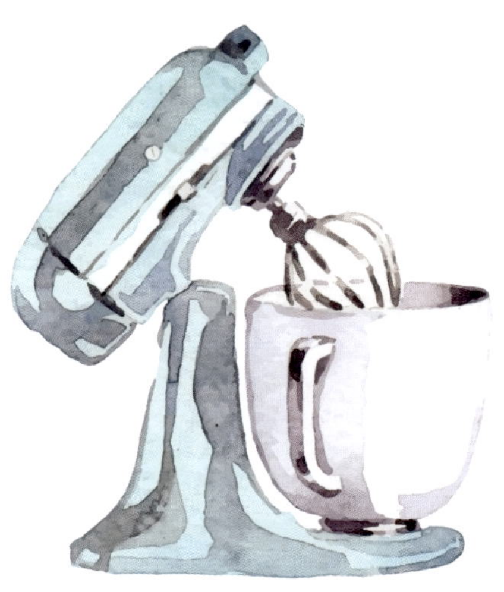

Remember the person you're taking care of as they want to be remembered: In their prime, at their best, having fun, helping you.

It won't always be like this.

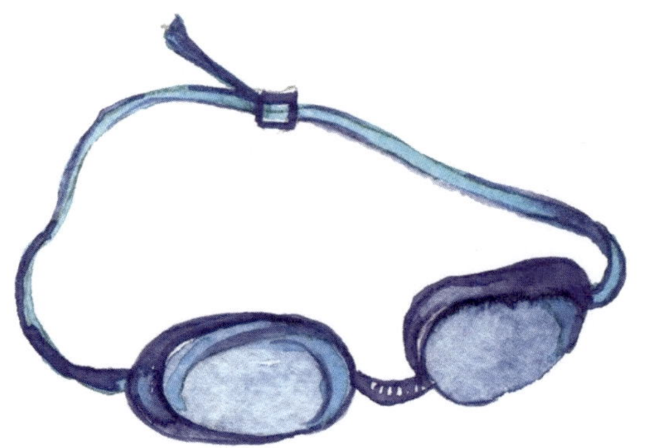

Check in with your body. Go on a walk, stretch, jump in a pool.

Reset your mind by resetting
your senses. Run your
hands under cold water,
or slide into a hot bath.

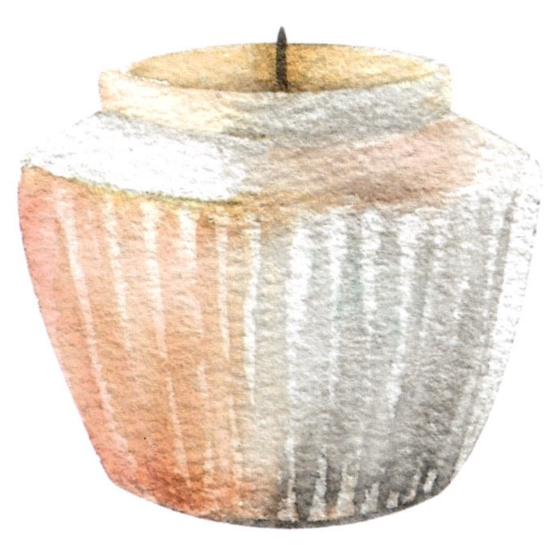

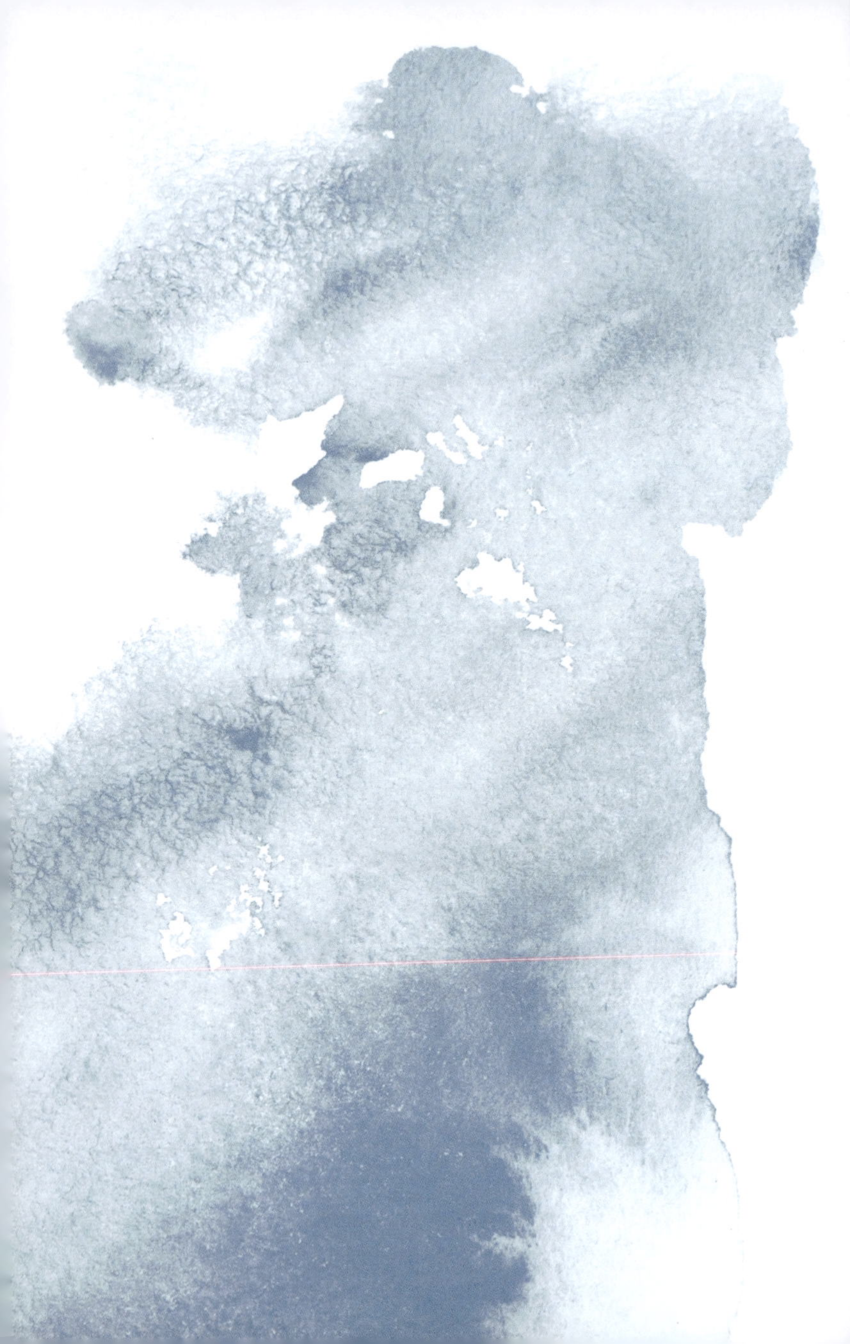

Seek out a support group for your person, too. Helping them find others who can relate to what they are experiencing might help them process their own feelings.

affirmation

SAY THIS OUT LOUD:

Mastering the art of
patience is a gift to myself
and my loved one.

“It is not the load that breaks you down. It’s the way you carry it.”

—attributed to Lena Horne

Find a trusted friend or family
member who will listen to you
vent without judging you.

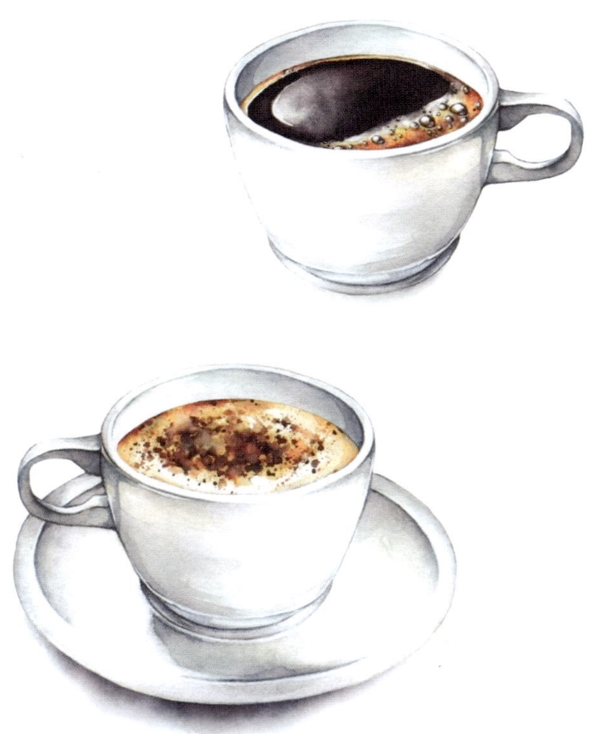

You are human. Some days will be harder on you than others.

It's important to find respite from your responsibility at times. Call on your person's trusted people to help you every once in a while.

"As you grow older, you will discover that you have two hands, one for helping yourself, the other for helping others."

—Audrey Hepburn

It's okay to set a boundary
about what you can and
cannot manage.

Have fun with your loved one.
Go down memory lane, watch
a fun TV show together, laugh.

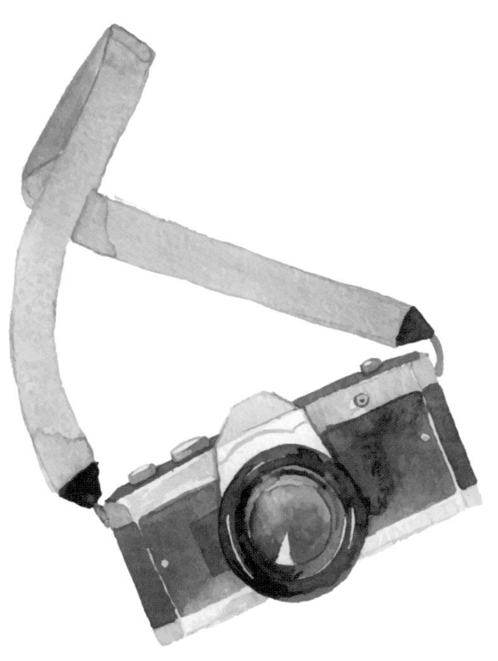

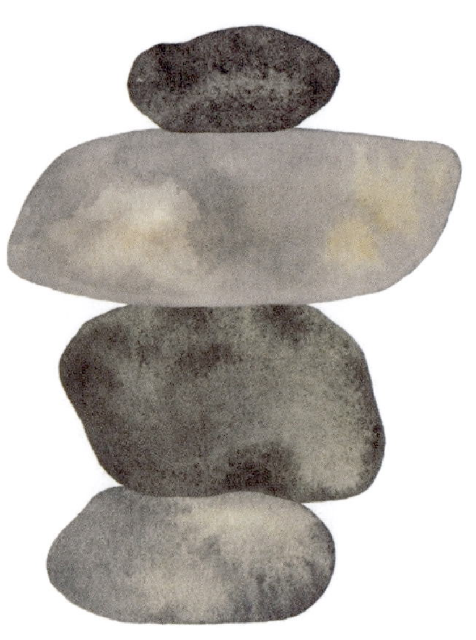

What can we give of ourselves
to our person? How can
we balance our worry with
the need to show up with
good energy for them?

It's important to think
about what you're capable of.
Centering the person who needs
care is at the root of our loving
connection as a caregiver, but
boundaries are important.

"You must do the thing you think you cannot do."

—Eleanor Roosevelt

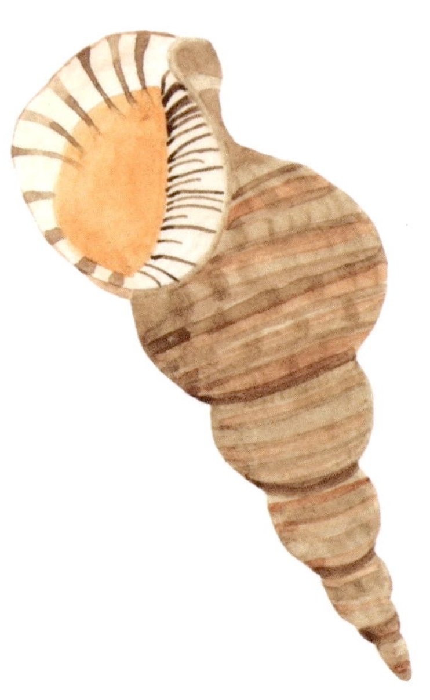

Close your eyes and visualize the most beautiful place you know. Try to experience it fully—imagine the sounds, recall the way it smells, and try to picture each feature of the landscape. Move through the space in your mind.

affirmation

SAY THIS OUT LOUD:

I am worthy of care and
support from others, and I
will ask for the help I need.

Listen.

Honor your person's wishes
as much as you can—they are the
center of this caregiving dance.

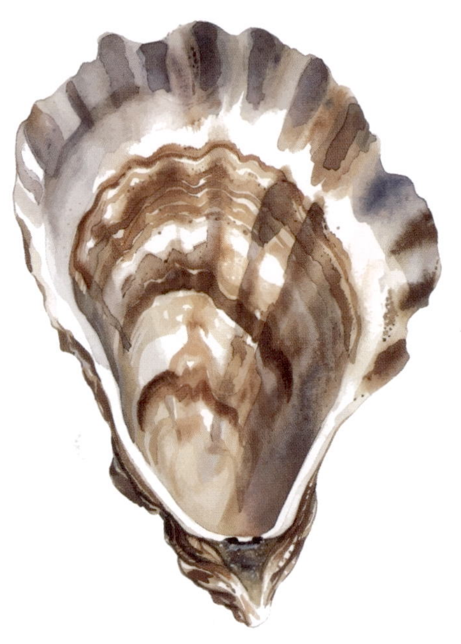

Lead with love, and usually
you can't go wrong.

RESOURCES

BOOKS

Still, I Rise: A Guide to Navigating the Caregiver Journey by Melody Vahcal, MS, CCC-SLP

The 36-Hour Day: A Family Guide to Caring for People Who Have Alzheimer Disease and Other Dementias by Nancy L. Mace, MA and Peter V. Rabins, MD, MPH

The In-Between: Unforgettable Encounters During Life's Final Moments by Hadley Vlahos, RN

Influencing Death: Reframing Dying for Better Living by Penny Hawkins Smith, RN

My Aging Parent Needs Help!: 7 Step Guide to Caregiving with No Regrets, More Compassion, and Going from Overwhelmed to Organized by Cynthia Kaye

When Your Child is Sick: A Guide to Navigating the Practical and Emotional Challenges of Caring for a Child Who Is Very Ill by Joanna Breyer

Being Mortal by Atul Gawande

APPS

Calm (for sleep, anxiety, and meditation)
www.calm.com

Headspace (for meditation)
www.headspace.com

WEBSITES

Caring Village
www.caringvillage.com

CaringBridge
www.caringbridge.org

ABOUT THE FOREWORD AUTHOR

BEVERLY E. THORN, PhD, is the author of *Before I Lose My Own Mind: Navigating Life as a Dementia Caregiver*, as well as hundreds of articles, two books, and four workbooks on coping with chronic illness. She spent decades as a faculty member at Ohio State University and the University of Alabama, where she went on to serve as director of the clinical psychology PhD program and department chair in psychology. Currently professor emerita, she is also a certified end-of-life doula and continues to publish, speak, and conduct workshops nationally and internationally on managing chronic illness.

The gift of self-care is important in all life stages—check out all the titles in the Little Book of Self-Care series:

A Little Book of Self-Care for Those Who Grieve

A Little Book of Self-Care for the College-Bound

A Little Book of Self-Care for Brides

A Little Book of Self-Care for Caregivers

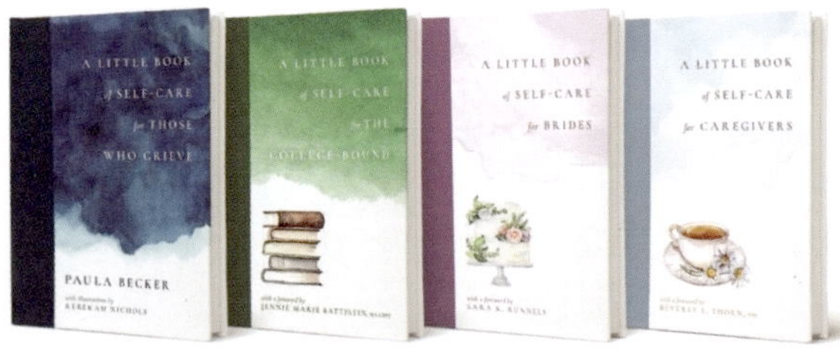